Meet Igor The Bad Leg Who Gave Me RSD

By

Pamela J Tomlinson

ISBN: 13: 978-1490367460

ISBN: 10: 1490367462

DEDICATION

I dedicate this book to my wonderful husband, who has supported me through Everything I have wanted to do. I dedicate this to my children who through everything we have went through in life my love is always there for you.

CONTENTS

ACKNOWLEDGMENTS

I acknowledge all the people out there with RSD
(Reflex Sympathetic Dystrophy) Anyone that might have a Igor living with
them that is causing them pain, this book is dedicated to you.

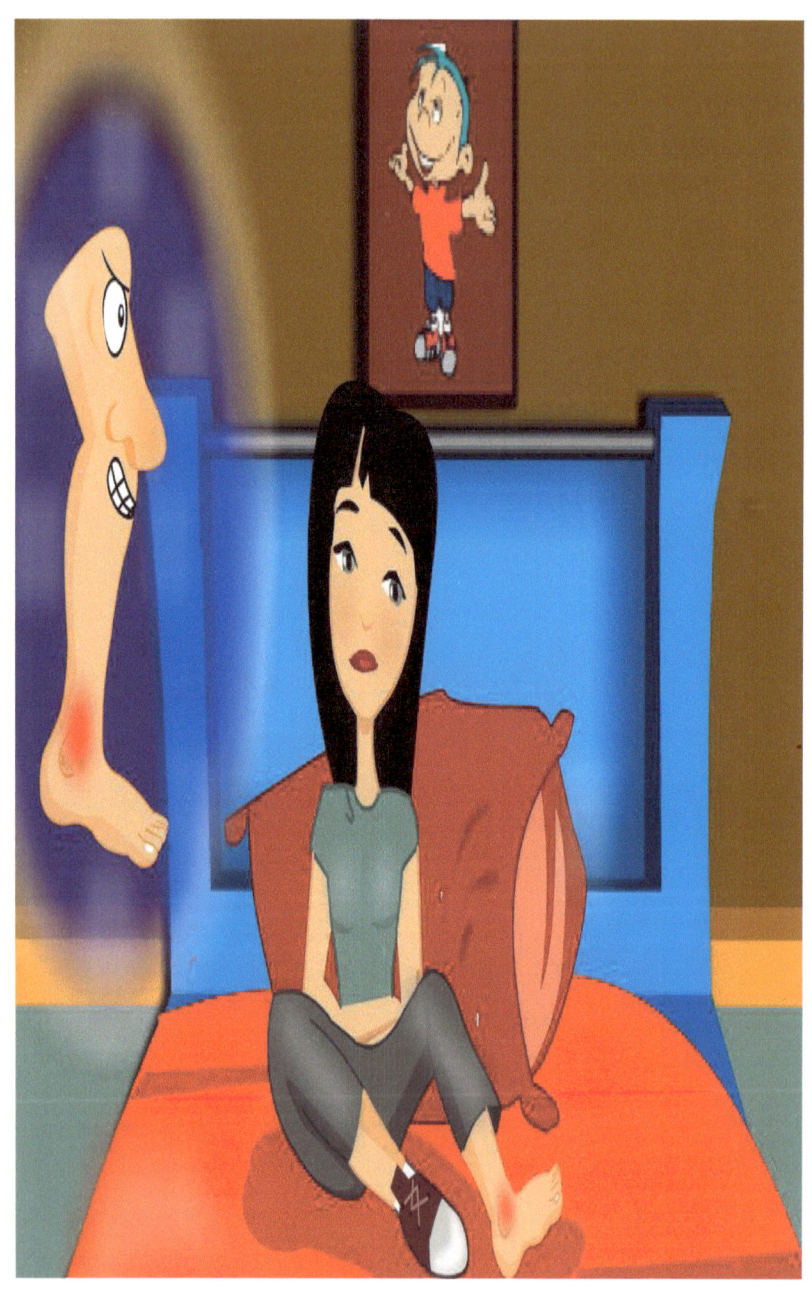

Igor is a bad bad leg
He likes to make me beg
At night he likes to make me suffer
He definitely is not a bluffer

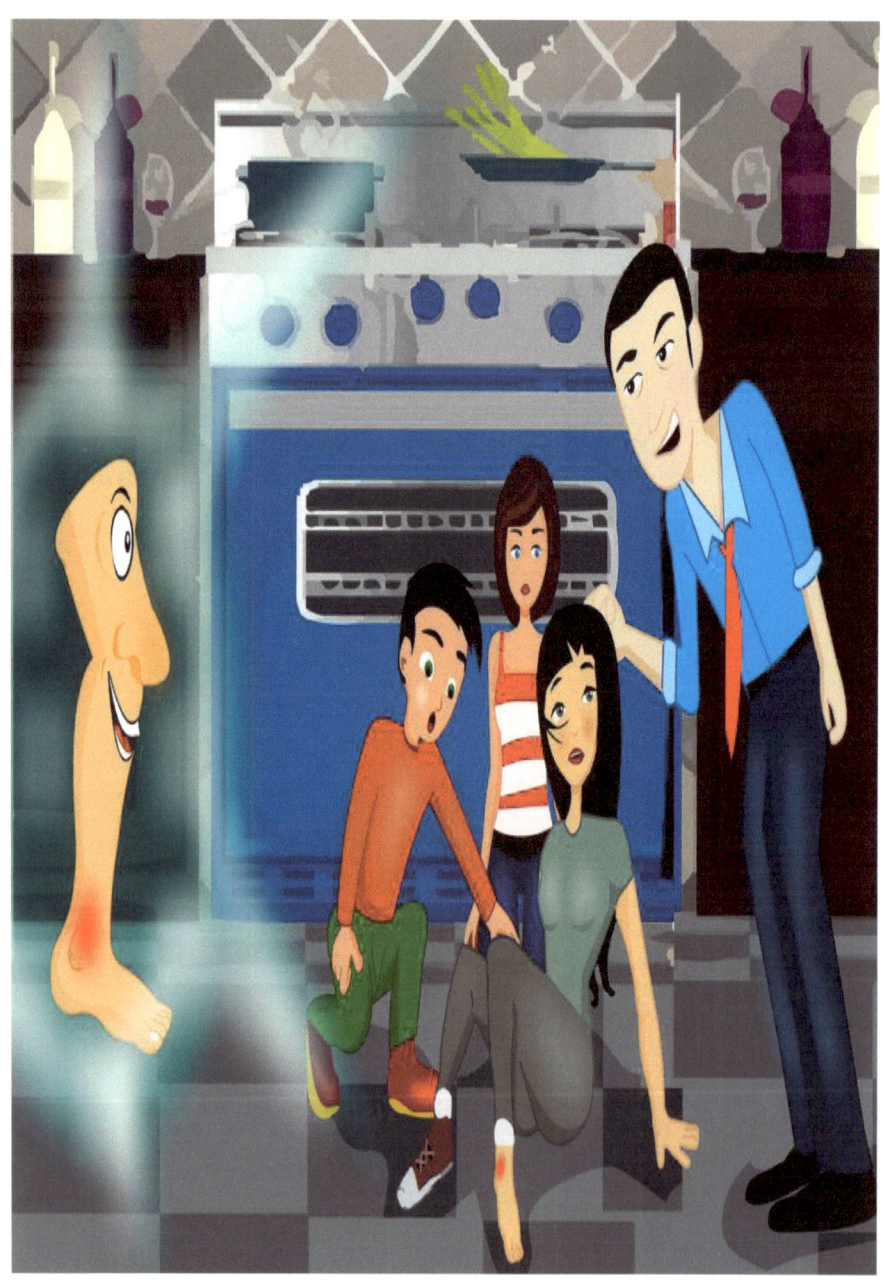

Igor came to live inside my leg
When I tripped one day on a peg
Igor is so mean to me
I am hoping one day he will flee

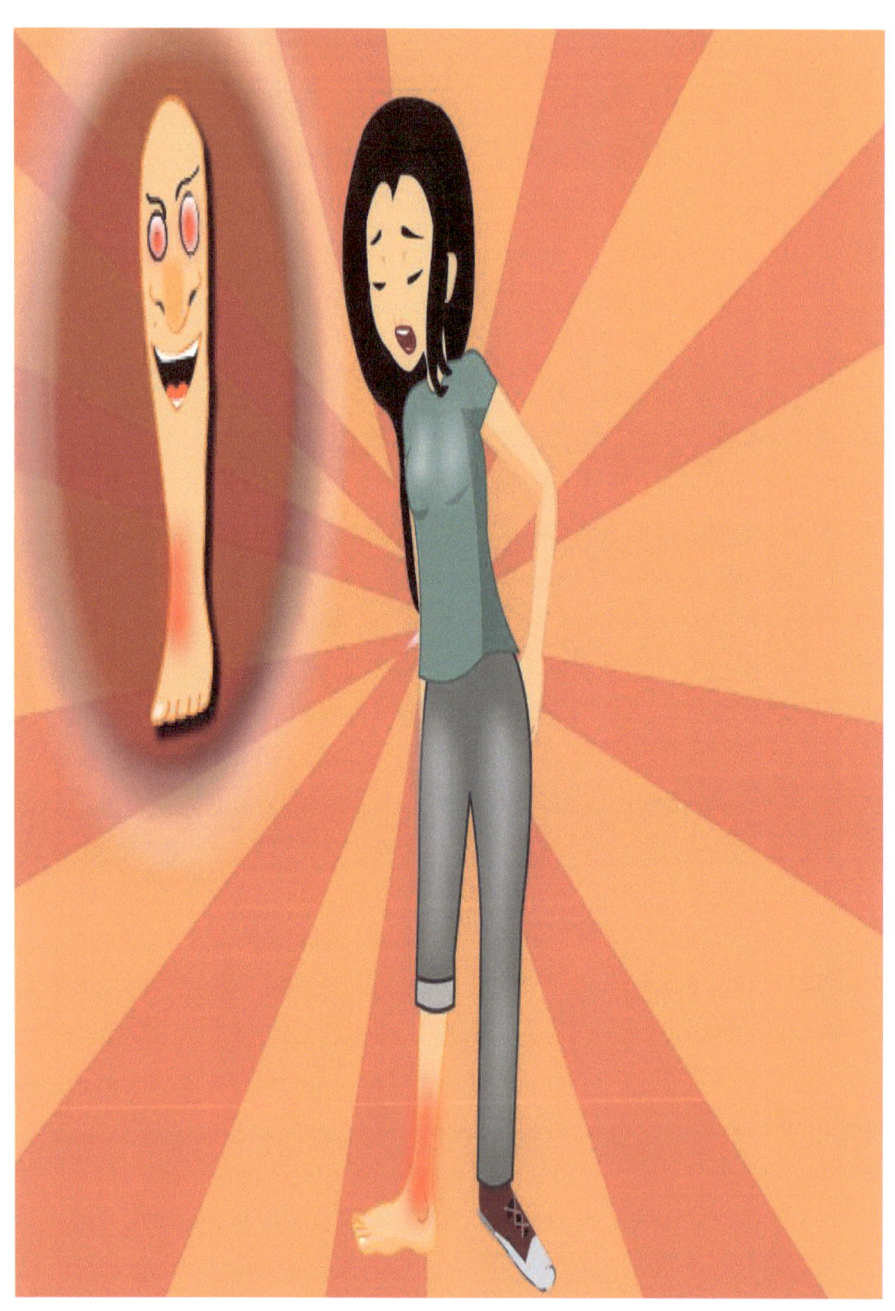

As long as Igor stays
He makes my leg feel like a blaze
Why does Igor have to be so mean
Igor is not looking so lean

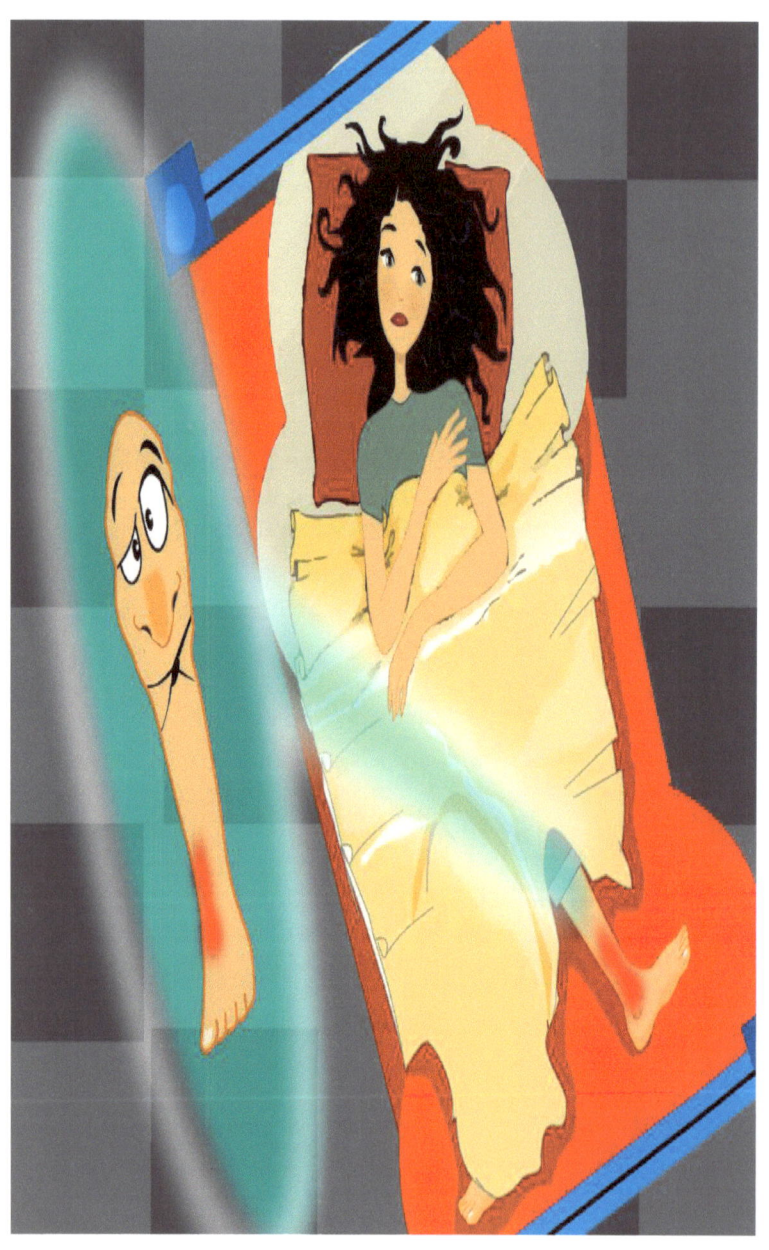

The longer Igor promotes RSD
The longer he is staying inside of me
Igor hates me most at night
He squeezed my leg oh so tight

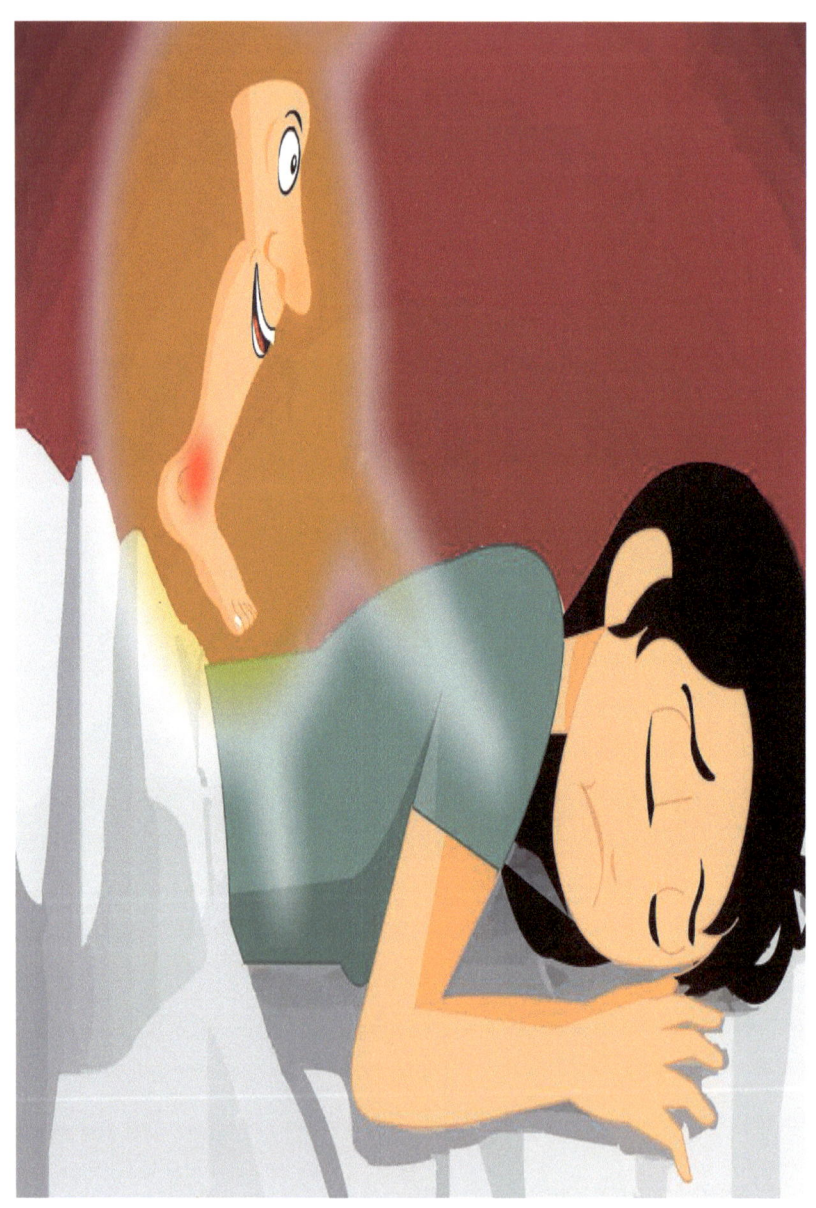

This causes me so little sleep
Nothing works, not even counting sheep
I hear Igor laughing at the pain he makes
With each passing moment of all the aches

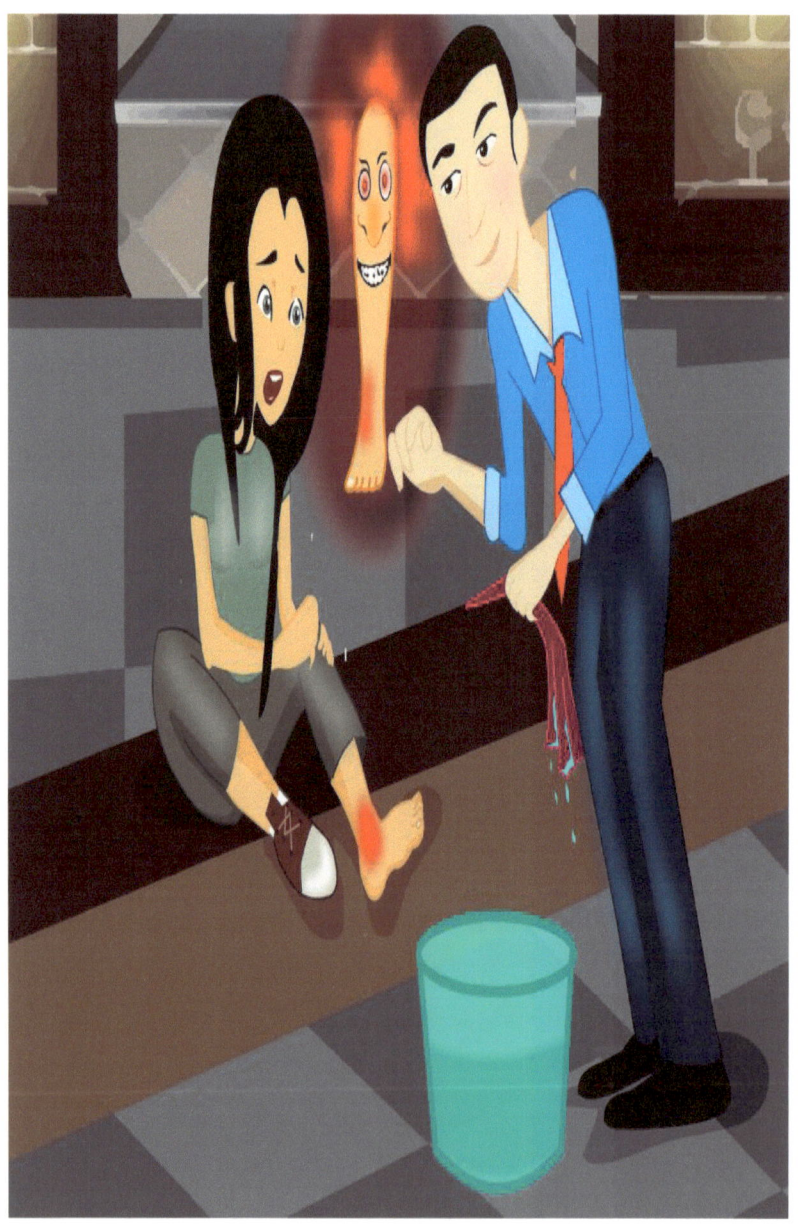

Igor will try to set my leg on fire
Igor is someone I do not admire
Igor why do you do this to me
Why don't you just get up and flee

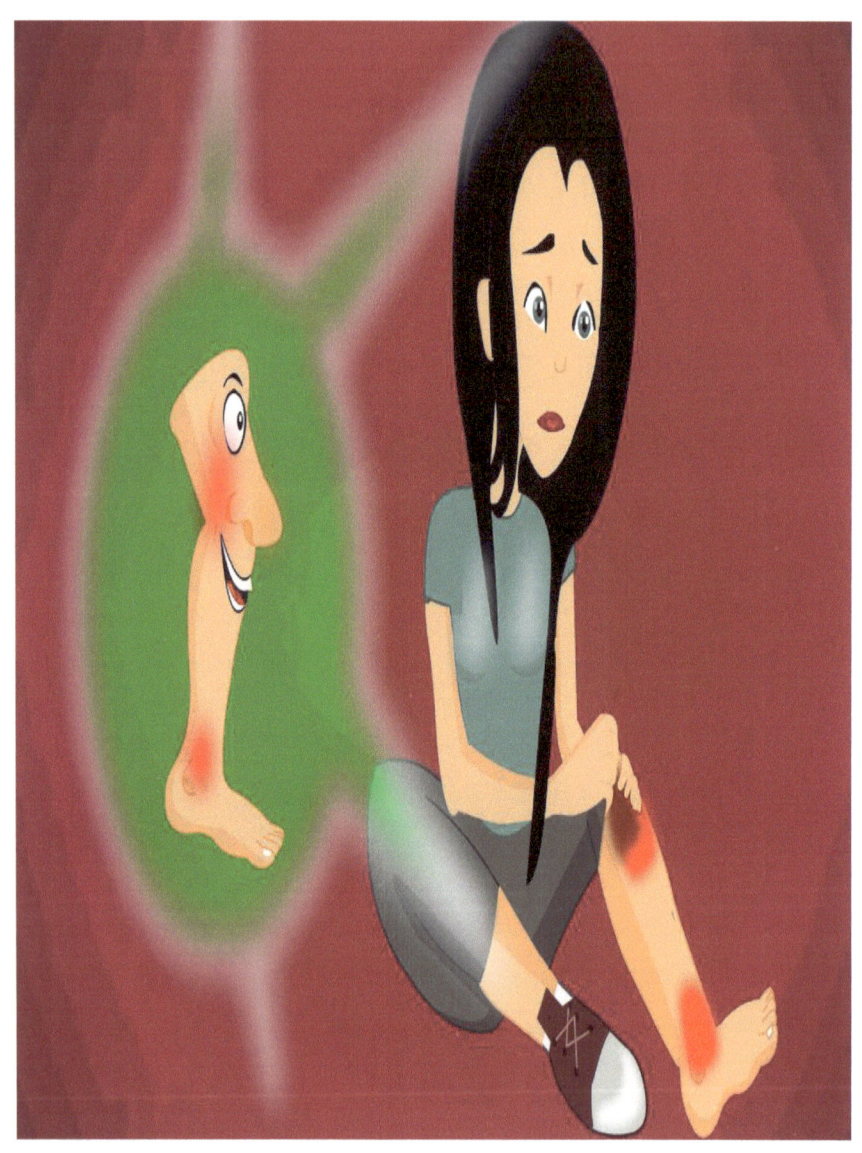

Igor will cause bruises on my leg out of the blue
There is so many not just a few
Igor will make my leg oh so big
When my leg used to look like a twig

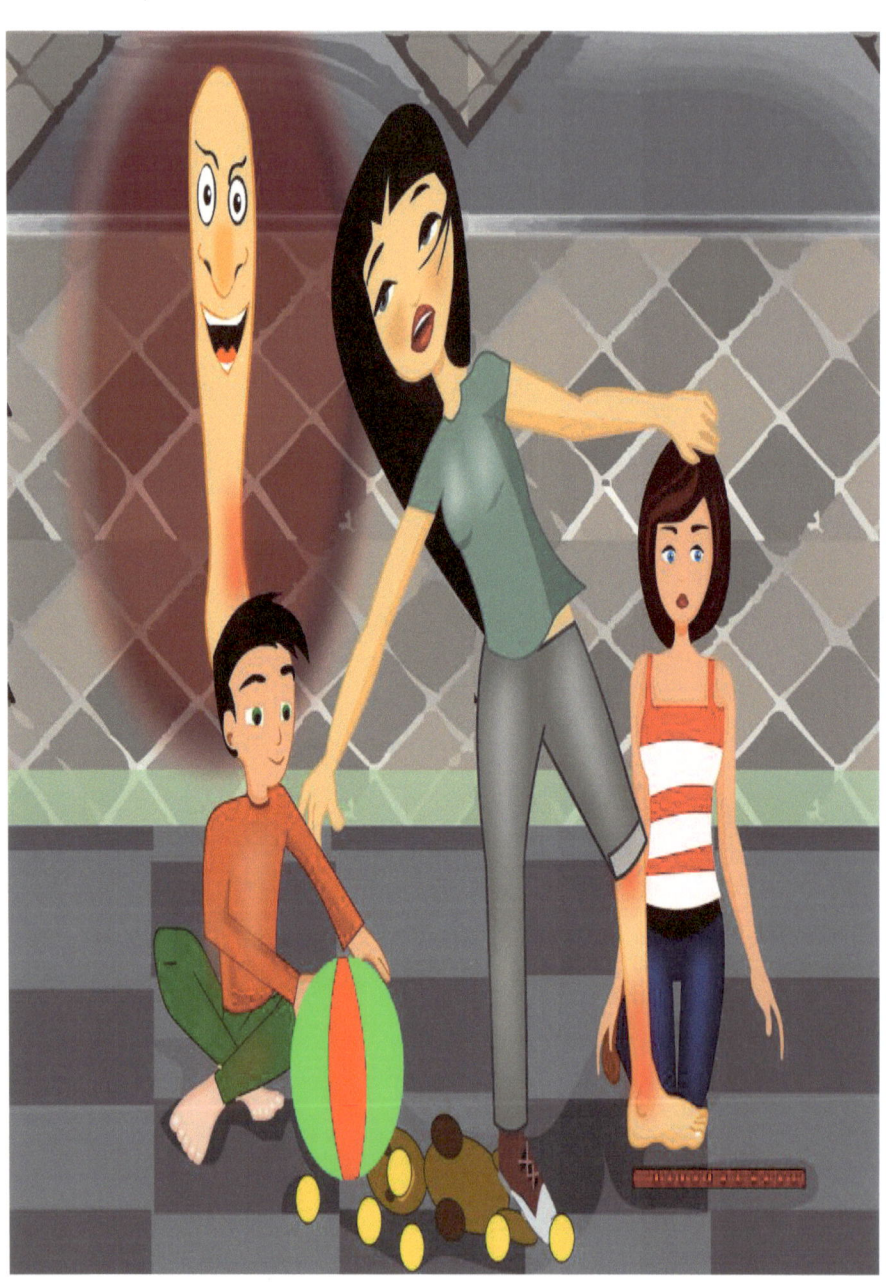

Igor will laugh at me if I bump my leg in pain
He makes me not want to think with my brain
Igor will make fun of the way I walk
He will try to get my leg not to work in shock

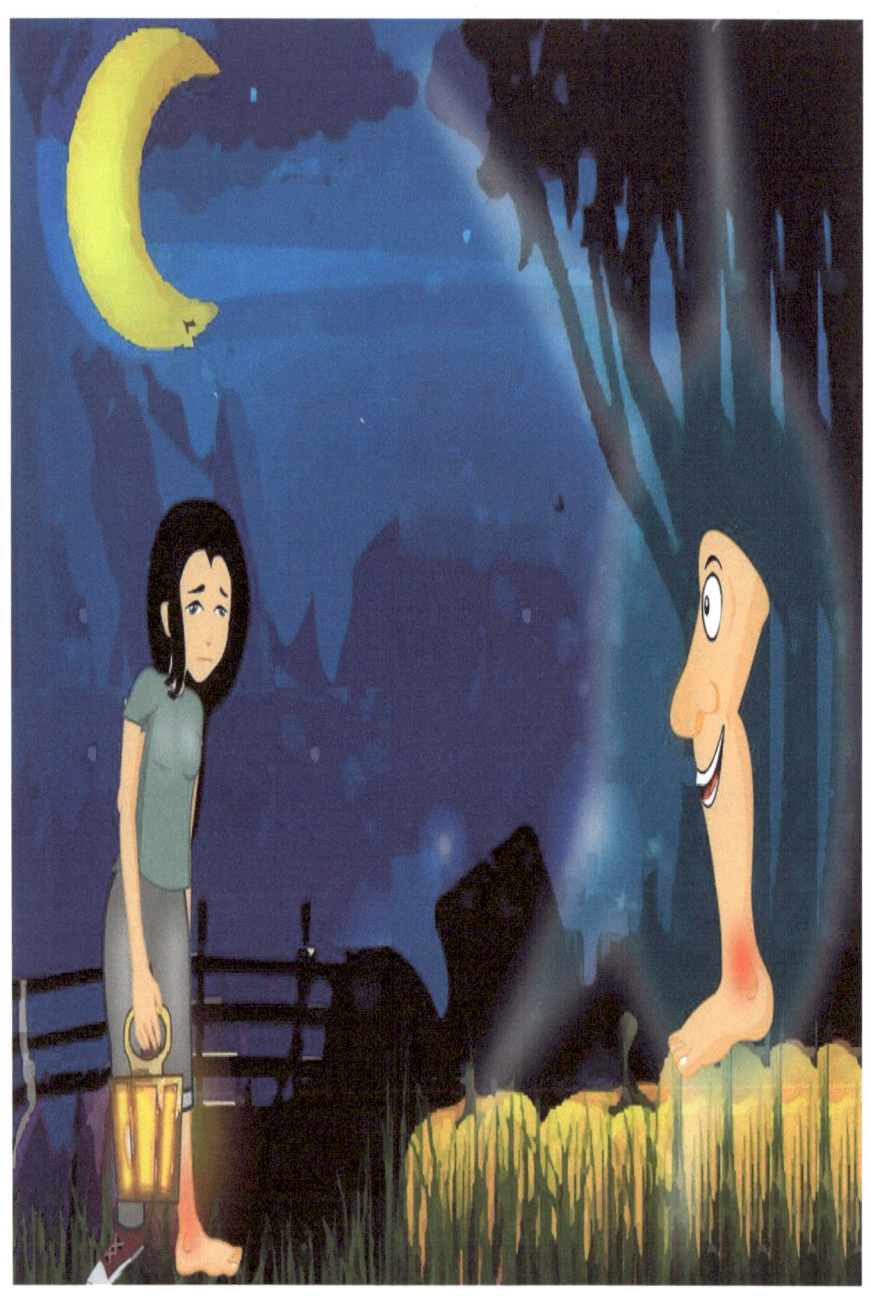

Igor will cause so much pain at night
My whole leg will want to yell in fright
Trying to get out of bed in pain
I have to reach for my cane

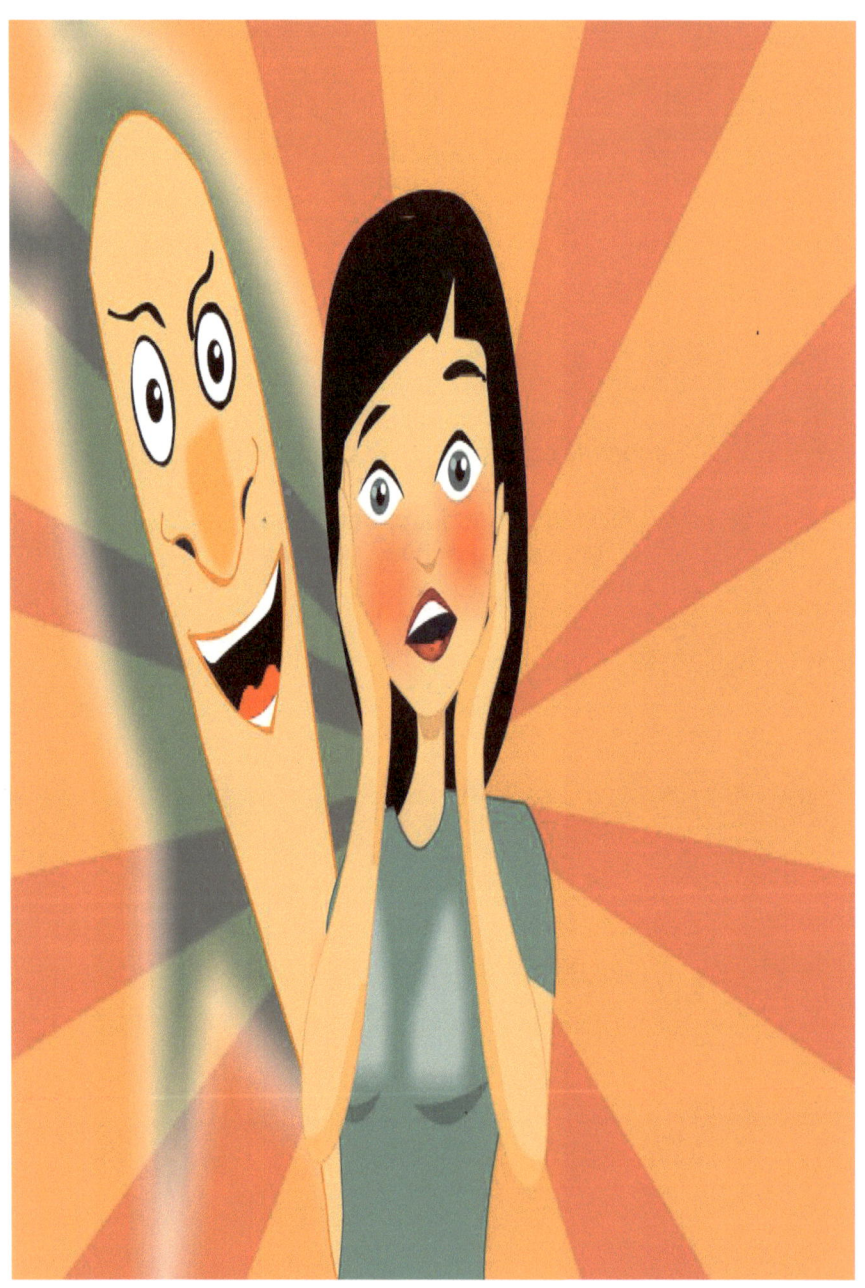

Igor makes me feel so bad
Then Igor makes me real mad
I really do not like Igor being so mean
Igor really does like to make a scene

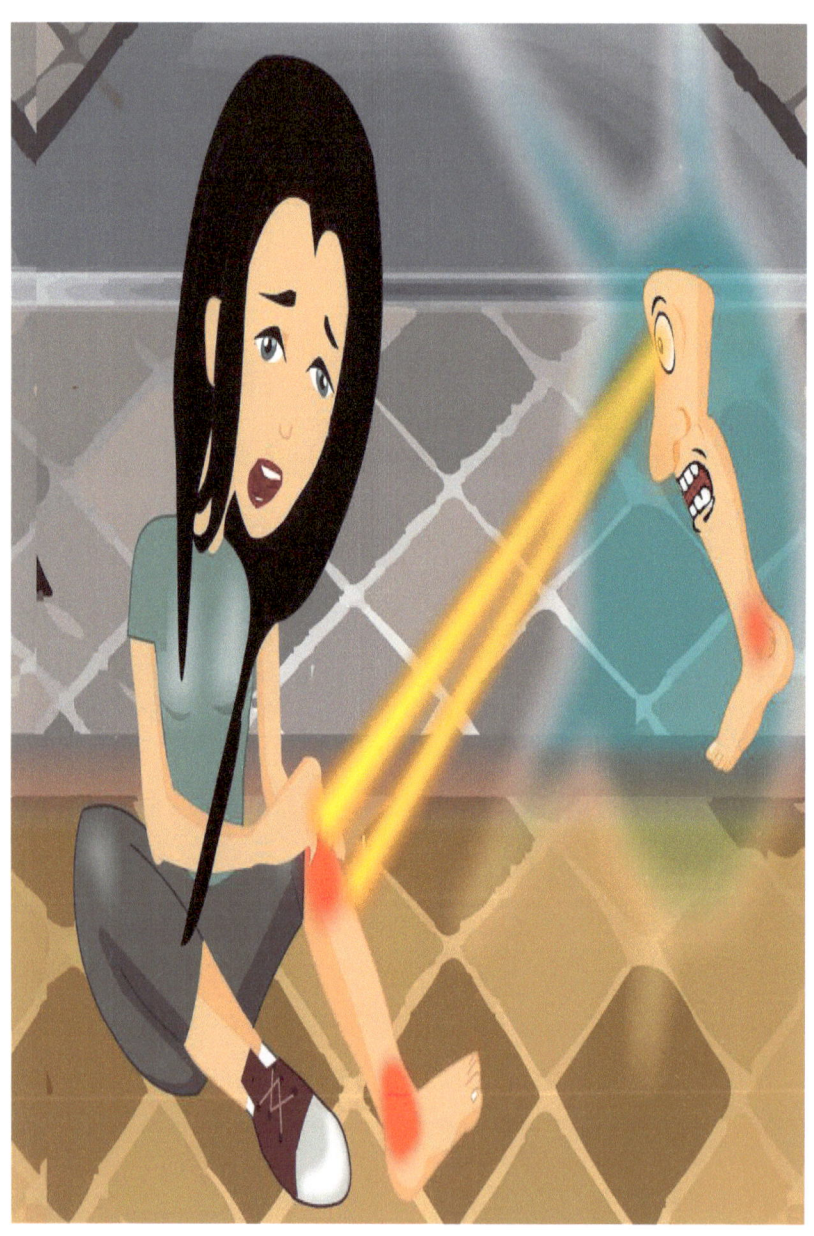

When getting out of bed so quick
Igor makes my RSD leg slick
The leg does not work to well
I fall to my face as I begin to yell

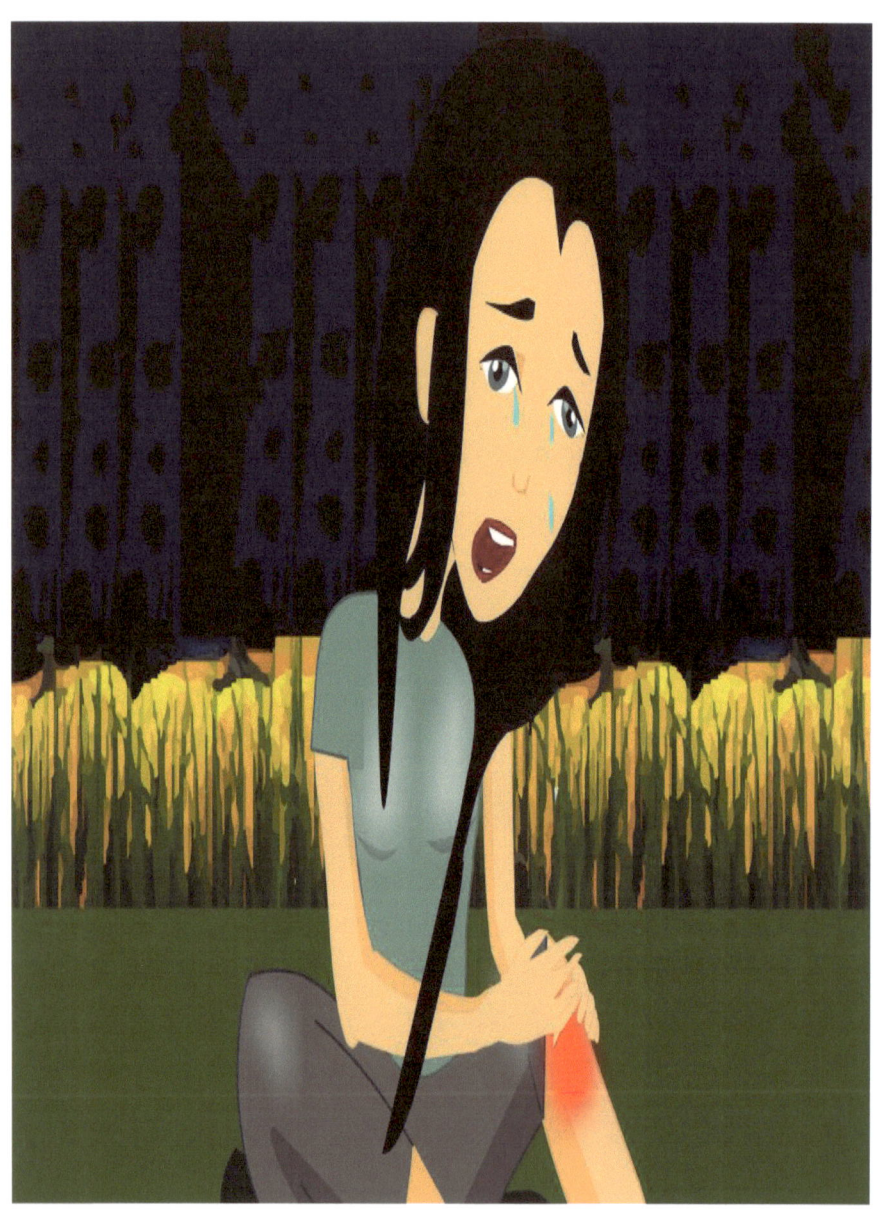

Even in the darkest of night
Igor is out there hiding causing my leg fright
He is lurking around the bend
He does not want my leg to mend

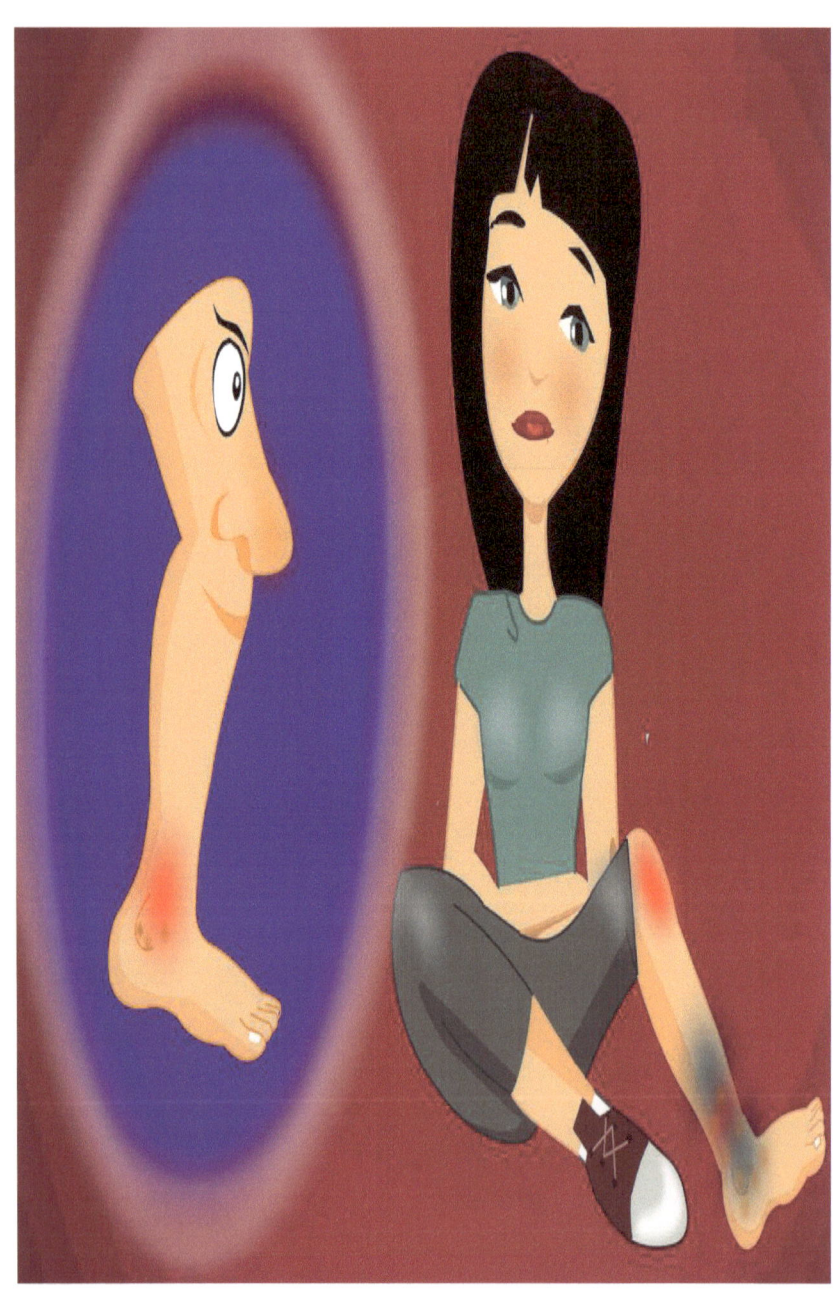

Igor makes my leg feel so hot
Makes my leg feel like it is in a knot
My leg will turn blue then will turn green
This really is not so keen

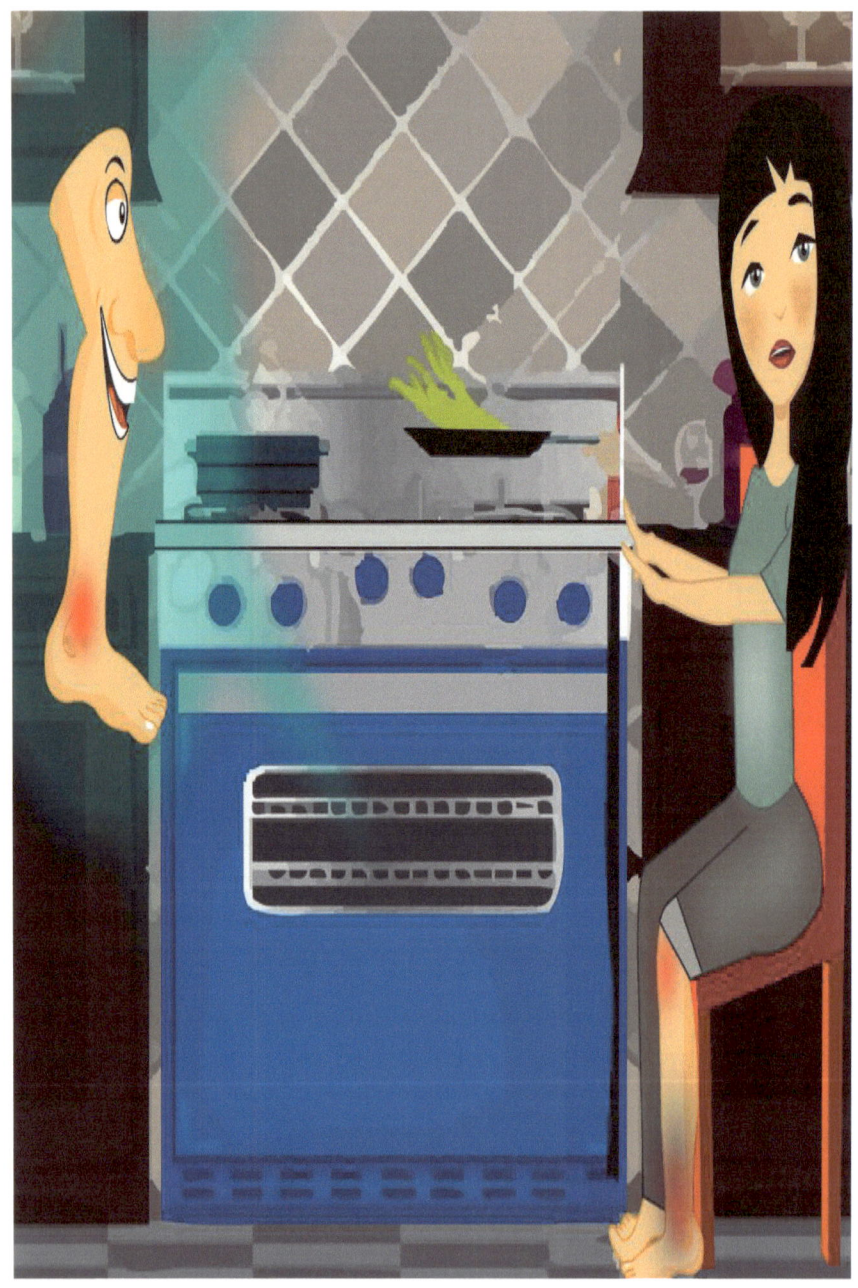

While cooking the dinner meal
My leg will hurt so bad I can not deal
I have to sit down on the chair
This really is not fair

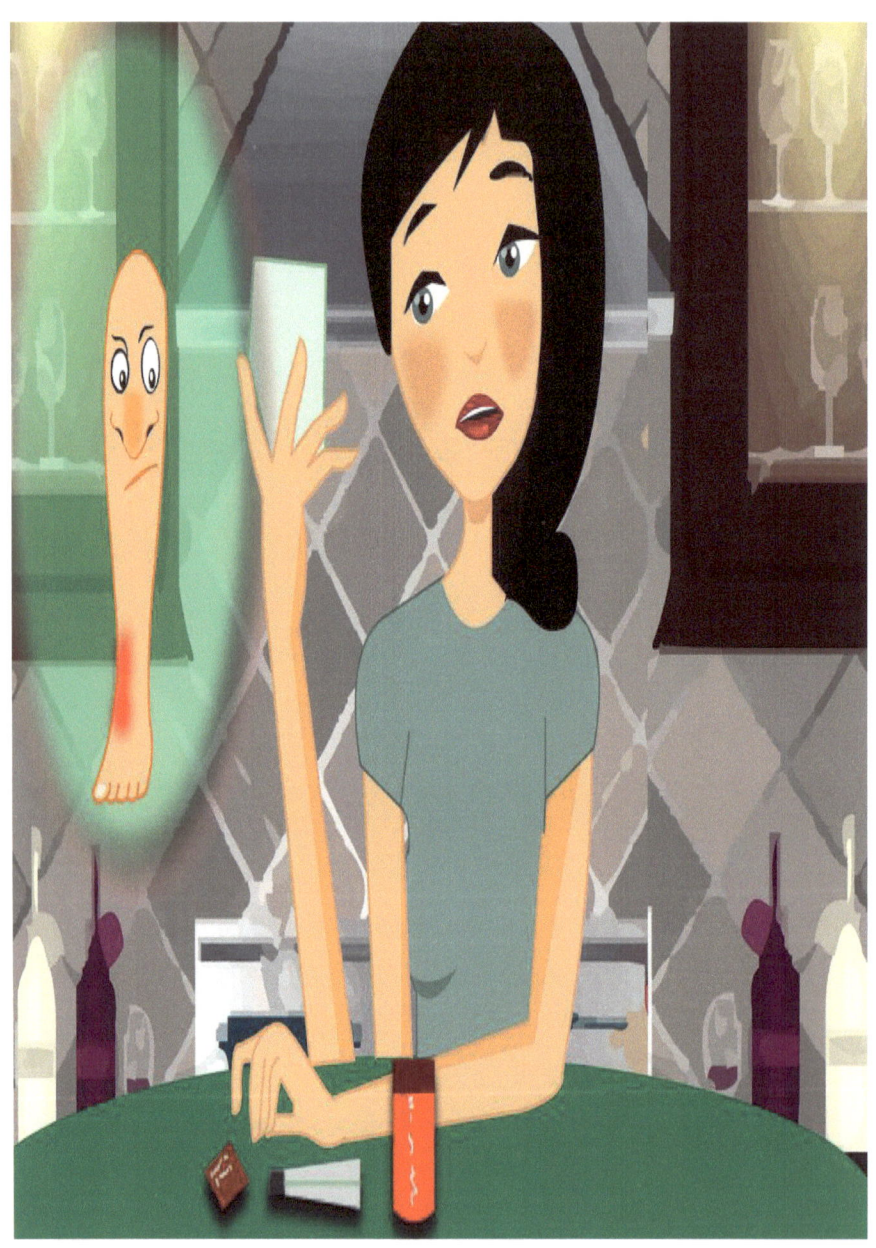

Igor you do this time after time
Why do you make this feel like a crime
You are taking away my everyday joys
It is hard to even enjoy everyday noise

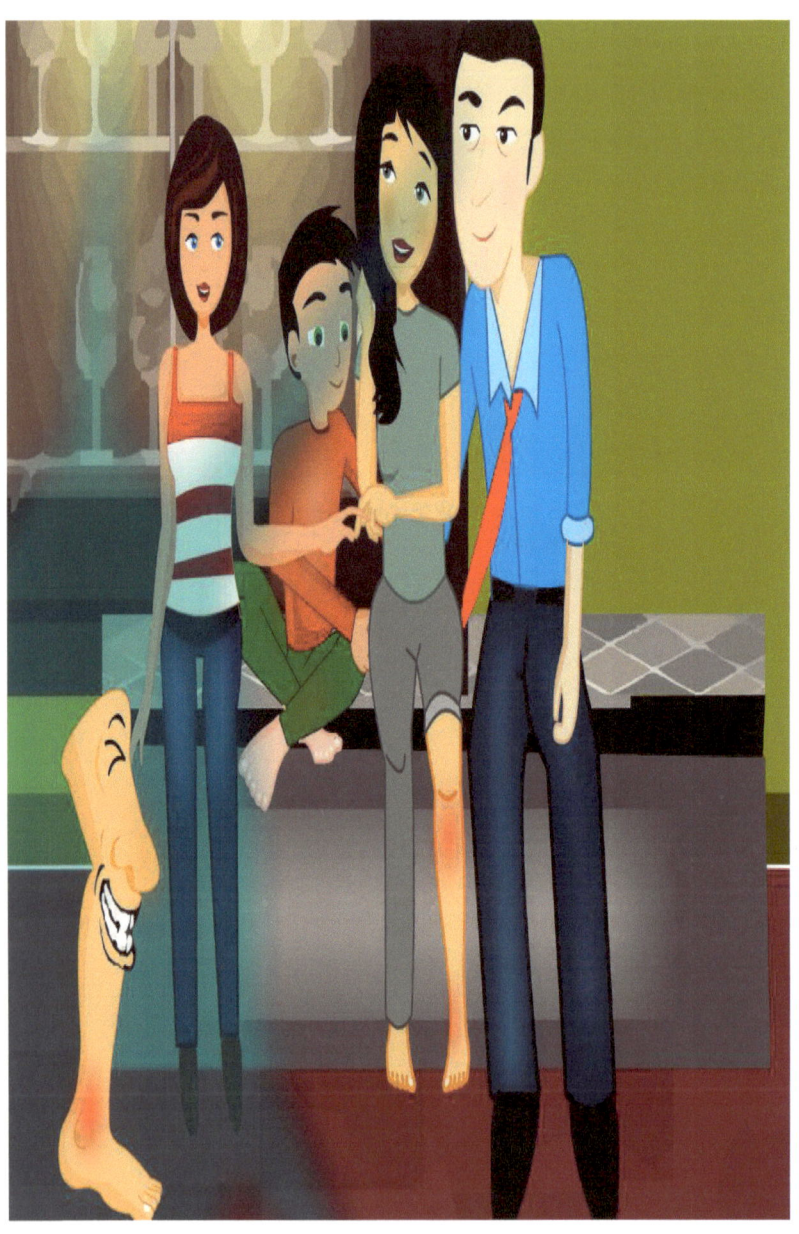

The littlest movement makes my leg ache
Igor makes my leg feel like a fake
Trying to find just the right spot
Hoping for pain free is a after thought

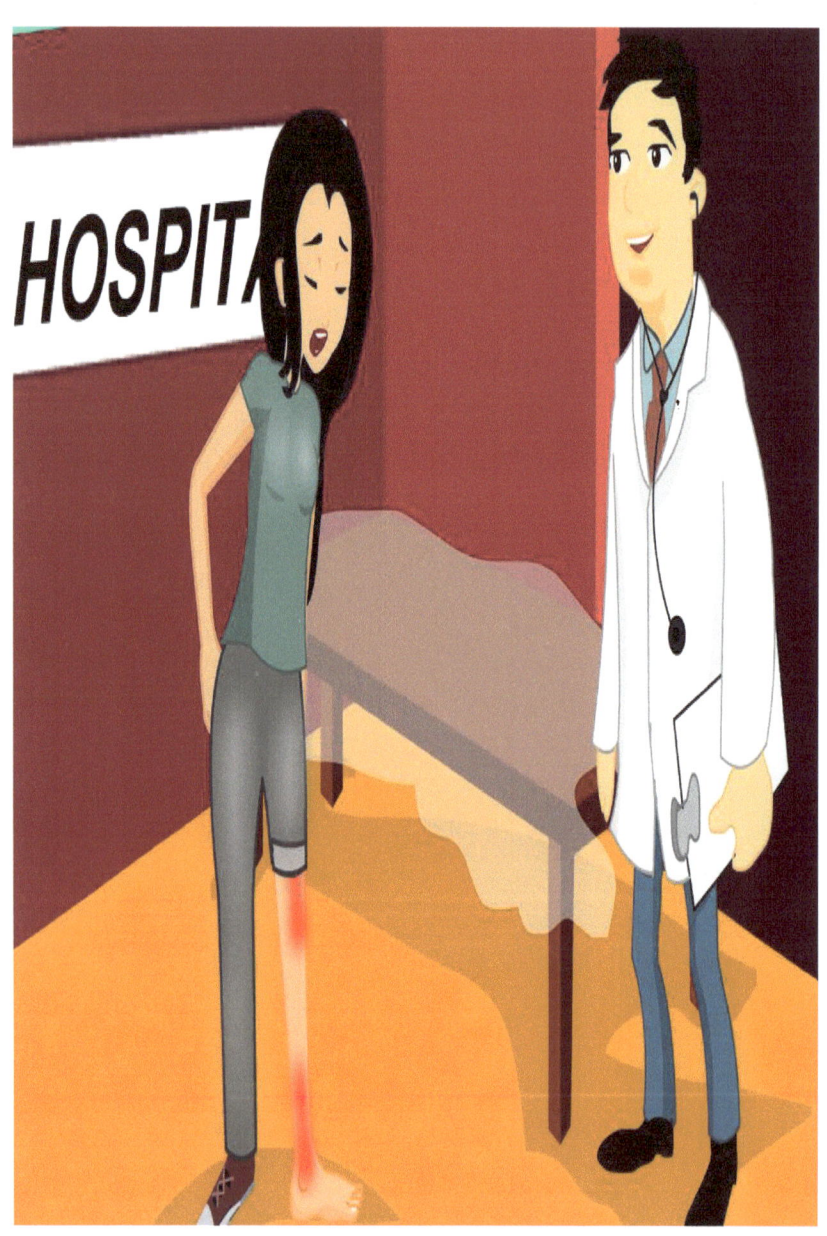

I can not even go for a simple walk
If I do it is back to the doc
Igor do you really enjoy these terrible games
Of making me feel like my leg is in flames

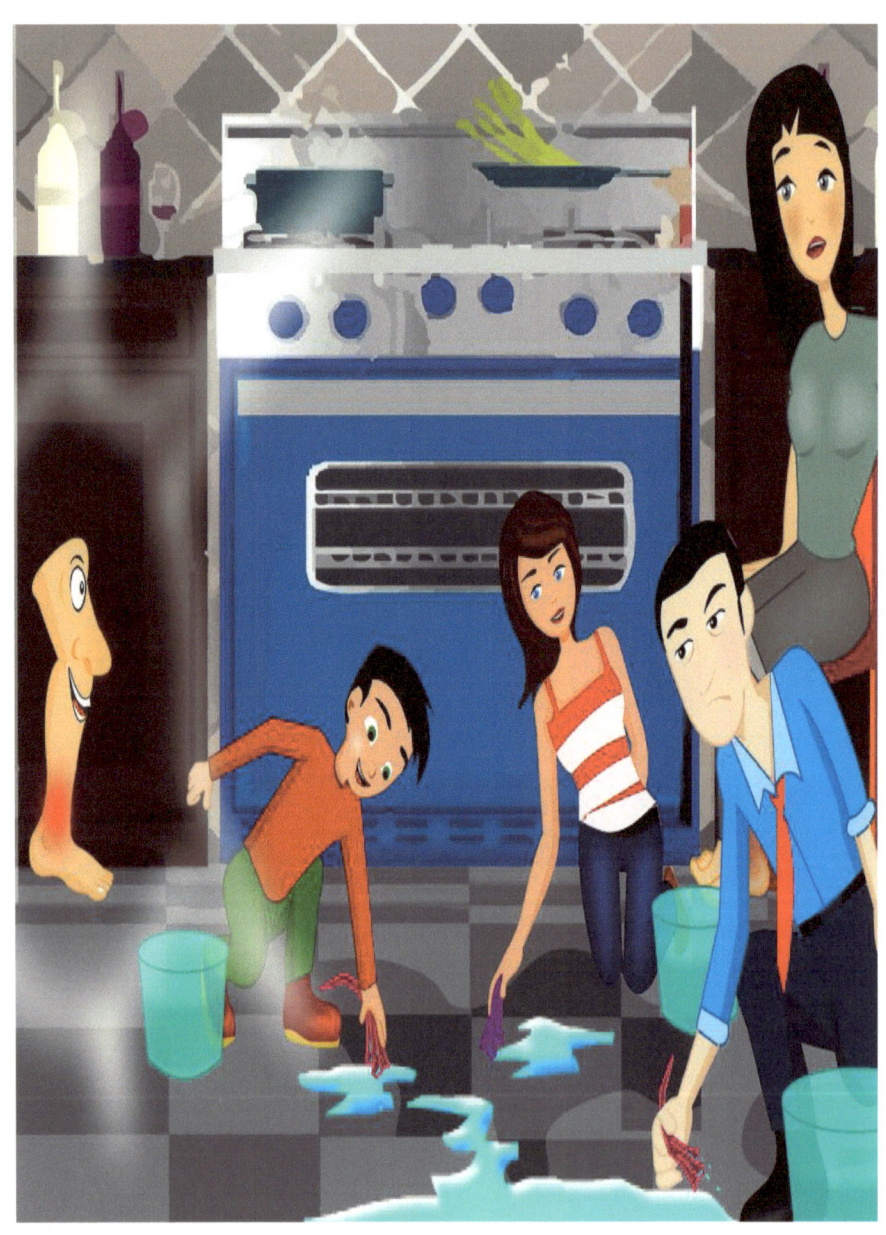

I can not even wash my own floors
Something as simple as doing my own chores
Igor please do not make me beg
Please give me back my own leg

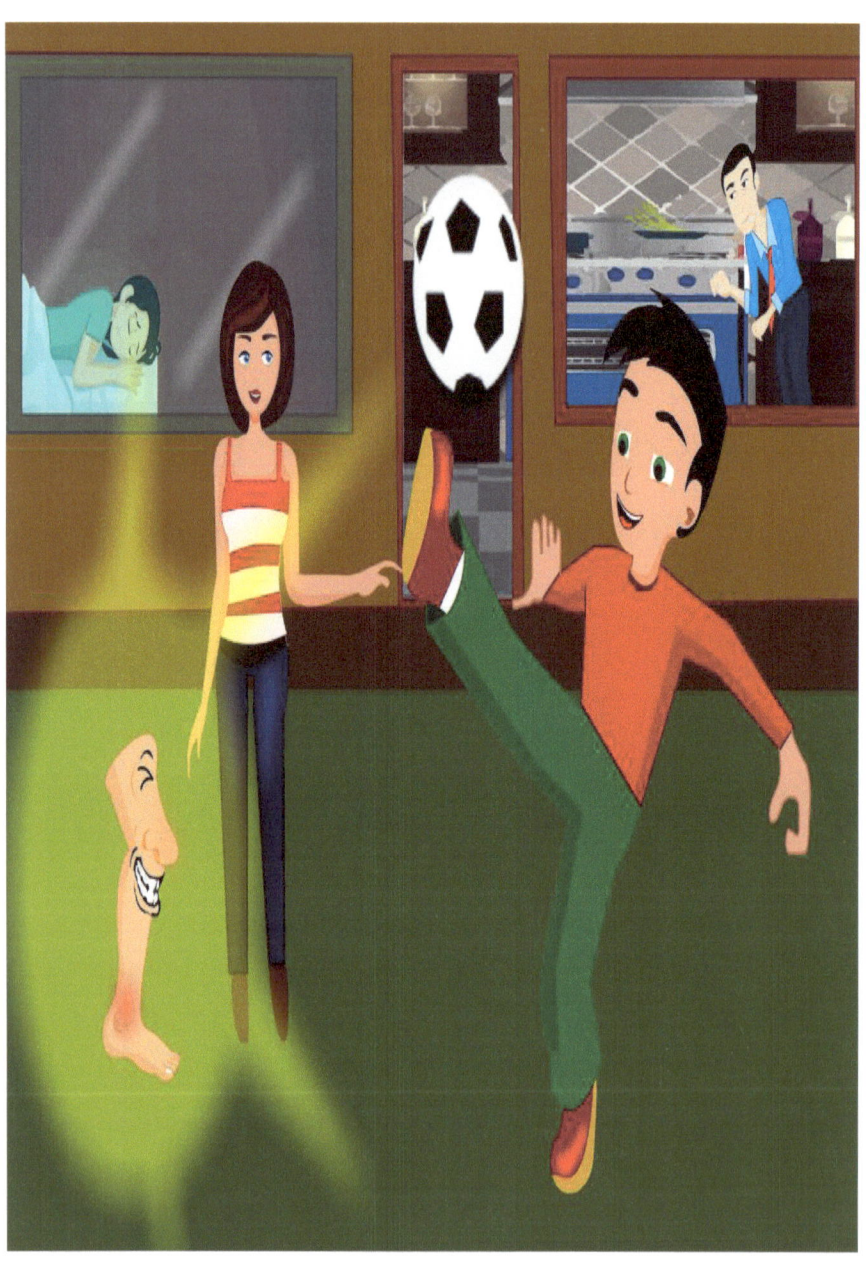

Igor said he is here to stay
My leg feels like a hunk of clay
If you have to be here all day
Once awhile go outside and play

ABOUT THE AUTHOR

Pamela J Tomlinson is a disabled/abled stay at home wife residing in Maryland who has the love and support and of her husband. Pamela J. Tomlinson is the founder of Kids Defense Team who brings awareness to a variety of adversities that children might need to overcome. Because of her disability she wanted to be a productive part of society by helping people in need. She goes by the Pay It Forward theory.

www.ingramcontent.com/pod-product-compliance
Lightning Source LLC
Chambersburg PA
CBHW040315010626
45792CB00022B/486